THE *Skinny*
NUTRiBULLET
LEAN BODY
ABS PLAN

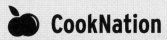
CookNation

THE SKINNY NUTRIBULLET LEAN BODY ABS PLAN
DELICIOUS CALORIE COUNTED SMOOTHIES & JUICES WITH CORE WORKOUT PLANS FOR GREAT ABS

ISBN 978-1-911219-34-7

A CIP catalogue record of this book is available from the British Library

• •

DISCLAIMER

This book is designed to provide information on smoothies and juices that can be made in the NUTRiBULLET appliance only, results may differ if alternative devices are used.

A basic level of fitness is required to perform the workouts in this book. Any health concerns should be discussed with a health professional before embarking on any of the exercises detailed.

The NutriBullet™ is a registered trademark of Homeland Housewares, LLC. Bell & Mackenzie Publishing is not affiliated with the owner of the trademark and is not an authorized distributor of the trademark owner's products or services.
This publication has not been prepared, approved, or licensed by NutriBullet ™ or Homeland Housewares, LLC.

Some recipes may contain nuts or traces of nuts. Those suffering from any allergies associated with nuts should avoid any recipes containing nuts or nut based oils.
This information is provided and sold with the knowledge that the publisher and author do not offer any legal or other professional advice.
In the case of a need for any such expertise consult with the appropriate professional.
This book does not contain all information available on the subject, and other sources of recipes are available.

This book has not been created to be specific to any individual's or NUTRiBULLET's requirements.
Every effort has been made to make this book as accurate as possible. However, there may be typographical and or content errors. Therefore, this book should serve only as a general guide and not as the ultimate source of subject information.

This book contains information that might be dated and is intended only to educate and entertain.

The author and publisher shall have no liability or responsibility to any person or entity regarding any loss or damage incurred, or alleged to have incurred, directly or indirectly, by the information contained in this book.

CONTENTS

NUTRIBLASTS UNDER 400 CALORIES

ABS PLAN WORKOUTS

OTHER COOKNATION TITLES

INTRODUCTION

The power of the Nutribullet, our delicious calorie counted smoothies and core workouts are a killer combination!

If you are reading this you will likely already have purchased a NUTRiBULLET or perhaps are considering buying one. A smart choice! The NUTRiBULLET is unquestionably one of the highest performing smoothie creators on the market. Its clean lines and compact design look great in any kitchen. It's simple to use, easy to clean and the results are amazing.

You may have watched or read some of the NUTRiBULLET marketing videos and literature which make claims of using the power of the NUTRiBULLET to help you lose weight, boost your immune system and fight a number of ailments and diseases. Of course the 'healing' power comes from the foods we use to make our smoothies but the real difference with the NUTRiBULLET is that it EXTRACTS all the goodness of the ingredients. Unlike many juicers and blenders, which leave behind valuable fibre, the NUTRiBULLET pulverises the food, breaking down their cell walls and unlocking the valuable nutrients so your body can absorb and use them.

You may have made your own smoothies in the past using a blender – you'll know even with a powerful device that there are often indigestible pieces of food left in your glass – not so with the NUTRiBULLET which uses 600 watts to breakdown every part of the food. The manufacturer calls it 'cyclonic action' running at 10,000 revolutions per minute but whatever the marketing jargon, the results speak for themselves.

The NUTRiBULLET is not a blender and not a juicer. It is a nutrient extractor, getting the very best from every ingredient you put in and delivering a nutrient packed smoothie called a 'Nutriblast'. Using the power of the NUTRiBULLET is an incredibly fast and efficient way of giving our bodies the goodness they need. Making the most of anti-oxidants to protect your cells, omega 3 fatty acids to help your joints, fibre to aid digestion and protein to build and repair muscles.

Just one nutrient packed Nutriblast a day can make a difference to the way you feel and it only takes seconds to make!

All our recipes make use of the tall cup of the NUTRiBULLET and the extractor blade. Feel free to experiment. Mixing your ingredients is fun and will help your create wonderful new combinations too. As a basic formula, work on 50% leafy greens 50% fruit, ¼ cup of seeds/nuts and water.

There has never been a better time to introduce health-boosting, weight reducing, well-being smoothies to your life. With a spiralling obesity epidemic in the western world which in turn is linked to a growing list of debilitating diseases and ailments including diabetes, high blood pressure, heart disease, high cholesterol, infertility, skin conditions and more, the future for many of us can look bleak. Combine this with the super-fast pace of modern life and we can be left feeling fatigued and lethargic, worsened by daily consumption of unhealthy foods.

The good news is that you have taken a positive step to improve your life. The power of the NUTRiBULLET, our delicious calorie counted smoothies and core workouts are a killer combination and will set you on the path to a leaner, fitter body.

THE ABS PLAN WORKOUTS

If you are new to regular exercise or haven't been active for some time then firstly congratulations on making a positive step to getting back into shape! Exercise is a great way to improve not just your body but also your mind. Not only can regular physical activity help prevent illness it can also bring clarity and focus to your everyday life. It can help you lose weight, get trim and keep you feeling better. There are many benefits to reap from regular exercise.

Before starting on our core workouts it is important to evaluate your basic level of fitness. If you have any major health concerns such as those listed below we recommend first seeking a health professionals advice.

- Heart disease
- Asthma or lung disease
- Type 1 or type 2 diabetes
- Kidney disease
- Arthritis

- Pain or discomfort in your chest
- Back pain
- Dizziness or lightheadedness
- Shortness of breath
- Ankle swelling

- Rapid heartbeat
- Smoker
- Overweight
- High blood pressure
- High Cholesterol

If you are or think you may be pregnant we do not recommend you undertake the core workouts.

Our core workouts should be combined with a healthy nutritional lifestyle, which is why the calorie counted NUTRiBULLET recipes in this book are the perfect partner. You should however not rely solely on our recipes as your daily nutritional intake. Physical and indeed everyday activities require energy to perform so we recommend a balanced diet of carbohydrates, protein and fat. Using a fitness tracker such as MyFitnessPal will help you achieve your daily nutritional needs.

When performing the core workouts start off slowly. Don't rush in and try to perform each repetition too aggressively. You are likely to not perform the drill correctly and might cause yourself injury. Take your time to correctly execute each move with correct form and then as you gain confidence you can increase the pace.

The great thing about our core workouts is that they can be done at home without any equipment whatsoever and only take up 15 minutes of your day. Sure your abominable area in particular is likely to be tender for a few days as your body gets used to the core crunching exercises, but if you persevere you will find that each workout becomes more manageable, then you can start to push your body to achieve more challenging repetitions and sets.

We have compiled 4 core workouts to perform which also include some cardiovascular exercises such as 'high knees' and 'jumping jacks' to bring your heart rate up. You should aim to do all 4 workouts within a 7 day period (1 per day) using the remaining 3 days to rest. Try to alternate where possible between training and rest days. it's important to remember that your abs are muscles and therefore need time to recover and grow so don't ignore the rest days Each workout lasts for approximately 15 minutes and a simple explanation with diagrams of how to correctly perform each exercise is provided.

Ab workouts will successfully strengthen your core muscles and can help with lower back issues. It is important to recognise however that ab exercises alone will not diminish the layer of fat the covers the abdominal area. Many people make the mistake of thinking that performing hundreds of crunches on a daily basis will deliver a 'washboard' core. If this is your goal then you also need to embark on intense levels of cardio and conditioning combined with a lower carb diet (avoiding fast digesting carbs like white potatoes, rice and sports drinks) to reduce your body fat to a (healthy) level that will make your core muscles more visible. Someone once said that "abs are made in the kitchen" and it goes without saying that any exercise plan whether intense or more manageable should also be coupled with a sensible, balanced and healthy diet. Again we recommend seeking a health professionals advise before following any weight loss and exercise program.

WORKOUT TIPS

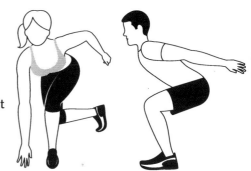

- Remember to breathe through each exercise
- Have a bottle of water to drink from between sets
- Always warm up and cool down before and after each workout
- Keep your core tight
- Enjoy!

NUTRIBULLET TIPS

To help make your Nutriblast fuss-free, follow these quick tips.

- Prepare your shopping list. Take some time to select which Nutriblasts you want to prepare in advance. As with all food shopping, make a note of all the ingredients and quantities you need. Depending on the ingredients it's best not to shop too far in advance to ensure you are getting the freshest produce available. We recommend buying organic produce whenever you can if your budget allows. Organic produce can give a better yield and flavour to your Nutriblast. Remember almost all fruit is fine to freeze too.
- Wash your fruit and veg before juicing. This needn't take up much time but all produce should be washed clean of any traces of bacteria, pesticides and insects.
- Cut up any produce that may not fit into the tall cup, but only do this just before making your smoothie to keep it as fresh as possible.
- Wash your Nutriblast parts immediately after juicing. As tempting as it may be to leave it till a little later you'll be glad you took the few minutes to rinse and wash before any residue has hardened.
- Substitute where you need to. If you can't source a particular ingredient, try another instead. More often than not you will find the use of a different fruit or veg makes a really interesting and delicious alternative. In our recipes we offer some advice on alternatives but have the confidence to make your own too!

- To save time prepare produce the night before for early morning Nutriblasts.
- Some Nutriblasts are sweeter than others and it's a fact that some of the leafy green drinks can take a little getting used to. Try drinking these with a straw, you'll find them easier to drink and enjoy.

IMPORTANT — WHAT NOT TO USE IN YOUR NUTRIBLASTS

The manufacturers of NUTRiBULLET are very clear on the following warning. While the joy of making Nutriblasts is using whole fruit and vegetables there are a few seeds and pits which should be removed. The following contain chemicals which can release cyanide into the body when ingested so do not use any of the following in your Nutriblasts:

- **Apple Seeds**
- **Cherry Pits**
- **Peach pits**
- **Apricot Pits**
- **Plum Pits**

CLEANING

Cleaning the NUTRiBULLET is thankfully very easy. The manufacturer gives clear guidelines on how best to do this but here's a recap:

- Make sure the NUTRiBULLET is unplugged before disassembling or cleaning.
- Set aside the power base and blade holders as these should not be used in a dishwasher.
- Use hot soapy water to clean the blades but do not immerse in boiling water as this can warp the plastic.
- Use a damp cloth to clean the power base.
- All cups and lids can be placed in a dishwasher.
- For stubborn marks inside the cup, fill the cup 2/3 full of warm soapy water and screw on the milling blade. Attach to the power base and run for 20-30 seconds.

WARNING:

Do not put your hands or any utensils near the moving blade. Always ensure the NUTRiBULLET is unplugged when assembling/disassembling or cleaning.

ABOUT 🍎 CookNation

CookNation is the leading publisher of innovative and practical recipe books for the modern, health conscious cook. CookNation titles bring together delicious, easy and practical recipes with their unique approach - easy and delicious, no-nonsense recipes - making cooking for diets and healthy eating fast, simple and fun.

With a range of #1 best-selling titles - from the innovative 'Skinny' calorie-counted series, to the 5:2 Diet Recipes collection - CookNation recipe books prove that 'Diet' can still mean 'Delicious'!

THE *Skinny*

NUTRiBULLET

LEAN BODY
ABS PLAN

NUTRIBLASTS UNDER 200 CALORIES

KALE & CHIA SEED SMOOTHIE

191 calories

Ingredients

POTASSIUM +

- 50g/2oz kale
- 1 banana
- 120ml/ ½ cup unsweetened almond milk
- 2 tsp chia seeds
- Water

Method

1 Rinse the ingredients well.

2 Cut any thick green stalks off the kale.

3 Peel the banana.

4 Add the kale, banana, milk & chia seeds to the NUTRiBULLET tall cup. Make sure the ingredients do not go past the MAX line on your machine.

5 Add a little water if needed to take it up to the MAX line.

6 Twist on the NUTRiBULLET blade and blend until smooth.

CHEF'S NOTE
Great for breakfast, the high protein chia seeds will help you feel fuller for longer.

CASHEW SPINACH SMOOTHIE

195 calories

Ingredients

- 50g/2oz spinach
- 200g/7oz melon flesh
- 125g/4oz apple
- 1 tbsp cashew nuts
- Water

Method

1 Rinse the ingredients well.

2 Cut any thick green stalks off the spinach.

3 Core the apple, don't bother peeling.

4 Add the spinach, melon, apple & cashew nuts to the NUTRiBULLET tall cup. Make sure the ingredients do not go past the MAX line on your machine.

5 Add water, again being careful not to exceed the MAX line.

6 Twist on the NUTRiBULLET blade and blend until smooth.

CHEF'S NOTE
Cashew nuts give a lovely smooth texture to this juice, you could also use almond milk instead of water for the base.

RASPBERRY ALMOND MILK SMOOTHIE

190 calories

Ingredients

HEART HEALTHY

- 50g/2oz spinach
- 125g/4oz raspberries
- 250ml/1 cup unsweetened almond milk
- Water

Method

1 Rinse the ingredients well.

2 Cut any thick green stalks off the spinach

3 Add the spinach, raspberries & almond milk to the NUTRiBULLET tall cup. Make sure the ingredients do not go past the MAX line on your machine.

4 Add a little water if needed to take it up to the MAX line.

5 Twist on the NUTRiBULLET blade and blend until smooth.

CHEF'S NOTE
Try soya milk in place of almond milk as an alternative.

CHIA SEED DETOX

186 calories

Ingredients

- 50g/2oz spinach
- 200g/7oz apples
- 3 tbsp lemon juice
- 1 tbsp chia seeds
- Water

Method

1 Rinse the ingredients well.

2 Cut any thick green stalks off the spinach

3 Core the apple, don't bother peeling.

4 Add the spinach, apple, chia seeds & lemon juice to the NUTRiBULLET tall cup. Make sure the ingredients do not go past the MAX line on your machine.

5 Add water, again being careful not to exceed the MAX line.

6 Twist on the NUTRiBULLET blade and blend until smooth.

CHEF'S NOTE
Adjust the lemon juice to suit your own taste.

APRICOT COCONUT WATER

178 calories

Ingredients

MINERAL RICH

- 50g/2oz shredded lettuce
- 125g/4oz carrots
- 175g/6oz fresh apricots
- 250ml/1 cup coconut water
- Water

Method

1 Rinse the ingredients well.

2 Top & tail the carrots, no need to peel.

3 Halve and stone the apricots.

4 Add the fruit, vegetables & coconut water to the NUTRiBULLET tall cup. Make sure the ingredients do not go past the MAX line on your machine.

5 Add a little water if needed to take it up to the MAX line.

6 Twist on the NUTRiBULLET blade and blend until smooth.

CHEF'S NOTE
Coconut water is a good source of B vitamins and potassium.

SPINACH CINNAMON JUICE

195 calories

Ingredients

- 75g/3oz spinach
- ½ banana
- 100g/3½oz apples

- 250ml/1 cup coconut water
- 1 tsp ground cinnamon
- Water

Method

1 Rinse the ingredients well.

2 Cut any thick green stalks off the spinach.

3 Core the apple and peel the banana.

4 Add the vegetables, fruit, coconut water & ground cinnamon to the NUTRiBULLET tall cup. Make sure the ingredients do not go past the MAX line on your machine.

5 Add a little water if needed to take it up to the MAX line.

6 Twist on the NUTRiBULLET blade and blend until smooth.

CHEF'S NOTE
Cinnamon has been used throughout the ages to treat everything from the common cold to muscle spasms.

SOYA & WHITE CABBAGE SMOOTHIE

196 calories

Ingredients

PROTEIN SOURCE →

- 75g/3oz shredded white cabbage
- 75g/3oz pears
- 250ml/1 cup soya milk
- Ice or water

Method

1 Rinse the ingredients well.

2 Core the pear.

3 Add the cabbage, pear & milk to the NUTRiBULLET tall cup. Make sure the ingredients do not go past the MAX line on your machine.

4 Add a little ice or water if needed to take it up to the MAX line.

5 Twist on the NUTRiBULLET blade and blend until smooth.

CHEF'S NOTE
Cabbage is a surprisingly good source of vitamin C.

STRAWBERRY ALMOND MILK

199 calories

Ingredients

- 50g/2oz strawberries
- 250ml/1 cup almond milk
- 1 banana
- Water

Method

1 Rinse well and remove the green tops from the strawberries.

2 Peel the banana.

3 Add the strawberries, milk & banana to the NUTRiBULLET tall cup. Make sure the ingredients do not go past the MAX line on your machine.

4 Add a little water if needed to take it up to the MAX line.

5 Twist on the NUTRiBULLET blade and blend until smooth.

CHEF'S NOTE
Add more strawberries if you want to increase the sweetness.

MANGO OAT SMOOTHIE

199 calories

Ingredients

DIETARY FIBRE

- 100g/3 ½oz orange
- 2cm/1 inch fresh root ginger
- 2 tbsp natural low-fat yogurt
- 75g/3oz mango
- 1 tbsp porridge oats
- 1 tsp ground cinnamon
- Water or ice

Method

1 Peel and de-seed the orange.

2 Peel and de-stone the mango.

3 Add all the ingredients to the NUTRiBULLET tall cup, finishing with water or ice to taste. Make sure the ingredients do not go past the MAX line on your machine.

4 Twist on the NUTRiBULLET blade and blend until smooth.

CHEF'S NOTE
Mango contains nutrients that strengthen the immune system and promote weight loss.

RED CITRUS JUICE

116 calories

Ingredients

- 40g/1½oz beetroot leaves
- 150g/5oz orange
- 75g/3oz raw beetroot
- 1 tbsp lemon
- Water

Method

1 Rinse the leaves and place in the NUTRiBULLET tall cup.

2 Peel & de-seed the orange, break into rough segments and add to the cup.

3 Peel and dice the beetroot and add it, along with the lemon juice.

4 Add water to taste, making sure the ingredients do not go past the MAX line on your machine.

5 Twist on the NUTRiBULLET blade and blend until smooth.

CHEF'S NOTE
Beetroot aids liver function.

SUPER GREEN CLEANSER

158
calories

Ingredients

- 2 celery stalks
- 300g/11oz cucumber
- 125g/4oz kale
- 225g/8oz spinach

- 1 tbsp fresh coriander
- 1 lemon
- 100g/3½oz apple
- Water or ice

Method

1 Rinse the ingredients well.

2 Cut any thick green stalks off the kale. Core the apple, don't bother peeling.

3 Peel and de-seed the lemon.

4 Add everything to the NUTRiBULLET tall cup. Finish with water, and ice if desired, making sure not to go past the MAX line on your machine.

5 Twist on the NUTRiBULLET blade and blend until smooth.

CHEF'S NOTE

Apples have long been used in traditional remedies for skin problems & anaemia.

YOGURT BERRY SMOOTHIE

147 calories

Ingredients

- 100g/3½oz kiwi fruit
- 75g/3oz mixed berries
- 2 tbsp low fat natural yogurt
- 1 tsp honey
- Water or ice

Method

1 Rinse the berries.

2 Peel the kiwi fruit, cut it in half and add to the tall cup. Add the yoghurt, berries and honey.

3 Make sure the ingredients do not go past the MAX line on your machine.

4 Add a little water or ice if needed to take it up to the MAX line.

5 Twist on the NUTRiBULLET blade and blend until smooth.

CHEF'S NOTE
Kiwi fruit helps flush out toxins from the colon.

PUMPKIN SEED & CRANBERRY JUICE

132 calories

Ingredients

OMEGA 3

- 125g/4oz cranberries
- 75g/3oz broccoli florets
- 1 tbsp chopped mint
- 1 tbsp pumpkin seeds
- Water

Method

1 Rinse the ingredients well.

2 Add the fruit, vegetables, mint & pumpkin seeds to the NUTRiBULLET tall cup. Make sure the ingredients do not go past the MAX line on your machine.

3 Add water, again being careful not to exceed the MAX line.

4 Twist on the NUTRiBULLET blade and blend until smooth.

CHEF'S NOTE
Cranberries are believed to have a positive effect on the human immune system.

CLASSIC CARROT JUICE

173 calories

Ingredients

VITAMIN C +

- 150g/5oz kiwi
- 200g/7oz carrots
- Water

Method

1 Rinse the ingredients well.

2 Peel the kiwis and slice.

3 Top & tail the carrots, no need to peel.

4 Add the sliced kiwi & carrots to the NUTRiBULLET tall cup. Make sure the ingredients do not go past the MAX line on your machine.

5 Add water, again being careful not to exceed the MAX line.

6 Twist on the NUTRiBULLET blade and blend until smooth.

CHEF'S NOTE
Kiwi fruits are packed with dietary fibre.

MINTED APPLE JUICE

148 calories

Ingredients

CALMING HERBS →

- 200g/7oz oranges
- 100g/3½oz apple
- 1 tbsp fresh mint leaves
- Water

Method

1 Rinse the ingredients well.

2 Peel and de-seed the oranges.

3 Core the apple, don't bother peeling.

4 Add the fruit & mint to the NUTRiBULLET tall cup. Make sure the ingredients do not go past the MAX line on your machine.

5 Add water, again being careful not to exceed the MAX line.

6 Twist on the NUTRiBULLET blade and blend until smooth.

CHEF'S NOTE
As well as tasting great, mint is a natural digestion aid.

APPLE & PEAR REFRESHER

195 calories

Ingredients

- 100g/3½oz apples
- 100g/3½oz pears
- 1 banana
- Water

Method

1 Rinse the ingredients well.

2 Core the apple & pear, don't bother peeling.

3 Peel the banana and break into 3 pieces.

4 Add all the fruit to the NUTRiBULLET tall cup. Make sure the ingredients do not go past the MAX line on your machine.

5 Add water, again being careful not to exceed the MAX line.

6 Twist on the NUTRiBULLET blade and blend until smooth.

CHEF'S NOTE
Sweet and simple this is a lovely refreshing smoothie.

GINGER BERRY BLASTER

160 calories

Ingredients

CLEANSING

- 50g/2oz watercress
- 150g/5oz blueberries
- 1 banana
- 2cm/1 inch peeled fresh ginger root
- Water

Method

1 Rinse the ingredients well.

2 Peel the banana.

3 Add the watercress, blueberries, banana & ginger to the NUTRiBULLET tall cup. Make sure the ingredients do not go past the MAX line on your machine.

4 Add water, again being careful not to exceed the MAX line.

5 Twist on the NUTRiBULLET blade and blend until smooth.

CHEF'S NOTE
Ginger contains gingerol, which has powerful medicinal properties.

CHOCOLATE CHERRY PROTEIN

192 calories

Ingredients

MUSCLE BUILDER

- 125g/4oz cherries
- 1 scoop chocolate protein powder
- 250ml/8½ floz water
- Ice

Method

1 Rinse and de-stone the cherries.

2 Mix the water and protein powder in the NUTRiBULLET tall cup.

3 Add the cherries and some ice. Make sure the ingredients do not go past the MAX line on your machine.

4 Twist on the NUTRiBULLET blade and blend until smooth.

CHEF'S NOTE
Protein is vital to muscle growth and tissue repair.

SERVES 1

CHIA SEED & PEACH SMOOTHIE

198 calories

Ingredients

MINERAL RICH

- 1 banana
- 125g/4oz peach
- 60g/2½oz strawberries
- 120ml/½ cup unsweetened almond milk
- 1 tbsp chia seeds
- Ice

Method

1 Rinse the peach and strawberries. Remove the green tops from the strawberries.

2 De-stone the peach but leave the skin on. Peel the banana and break into three pieces

3 Add the fruit and chia seeds to the NUTRiBULLET tall cup. Pour in the almond milk and add ice to taste. Make sure the ingredients do not go past the MAX line on your machine.

4 Twist on the NUTRiBULLET blade and blend until smooth.

CHEF'S NOTE
Chia seeds are an excellent source of omega-3 fatty acids.

SOYA MELON SMOOTHIE

193 calories

Ingredients

- 200g/7oz honeydew melon
- 250ml/1 cup unsweetened soya milk
- 1 tsp honey
- Ice

Method

1 Peel, deseed & roughly cube the melon. Place in the NUTRiBULLET tall cup.

2 Add the almond milk, honey and ice, making sure the ingredients do not go past the MAX line on your machine.

3 Twist on the NUTRiBULLET blade and blend until smooth.

CHEF'S NOTE

Try also with other types of melon, such as Galia and Cantaloupe.

THE *Skinny*

NUTRiBULLET

LEAN BODY
ABS PLAN

NUTRIBLASTS UNDER 300 CALORIES

STRAWBERRY ALMOND MILK

272 calories

Ingredients

NUTTY GOODNESS

- 150g/5oz strawberries
- 1 banana
- 250ml/1 cup unsweetened almond milk
- 1 tbsp almonds
- Water

Method

1 Rinse the ingredients well.

2 Remove any green tops from the strawberries.

3 Peel the banana.

4 Add the fruit, milk & almonds to the NUTRiBULLET tall cup. Make sure the ingredients do not go past the MAX line on your machine.

5 Add a little water if needed to take it up to the MAX line.

6 Twist on the NUTRiBULLET blade and blend until smooth.

CHEF'S NOTE
Use almonds which still have their skins on as the antioxidants are concentrated in this outer layer.

BLACKBERRY GREEK YOGURT SMOOTHIE

245 calories

Ingredients

- 125g/4oz blackberries
- 1 banana
- 150g/5oz apple
- 3 tbsp low fat Greek yogurt
- Water

Method

1 Rinse the blackcurrants.

2 Peel the banana and break into three pieces. Core the apple, don't bother peeling.

3 Add everything to the NUTRiBULLET tall cup. Make sure the ingredients do not go past the MAX line on your machine.

4 Add a little water if needed to take it up to the MAX line.

5 Twist on the NUTRiBULLET blade and blend until smooth.

CHEF'S NOTE
Greek yogurt provides a lovely thick base to this smoothie.

NATURALLY SWEET APPLE JUICE

232 calories

Ingredients

FLAVONOIDS

- 50g/2oz spinach
- 250g/9oz apple
- 1 banana
- 2 tsp honey
- Water

Method

1 Rinse the ingredients well.

2 Remove any thick stalks from the spinach.

3 Core the apple and peel the banana.

4 Add the spinach, fruit & honey to the NUTRiBULLET tall cup. Make sure the ingredients do not go past the MAX line on your machine.

5 Add water, again being careful not to exceed the MAX line.

6 Twist on the NUTRiBULLET blade and blend until smooth.

CHEF'S NOTE

Never use cooking apples for smoothies. Their taste it too sharp.

GOJI GOODNESS

270 calories

Ingredients

- 50g/2oz spinach
- 1 banana
- 370ml/1½ cups unsweetened almond milk
- 3 tbsp goji berries
- Water

Method

1 Rinse the ingredients well.

2 Remove any thick stalks from the spinach.

3 Peel the banana.

4 Add the spinach, banana, almond milk & goji berries to the NUTRiBULLET tall cup. Make sure the ingredients do not go past the MAX line on your machine.

5 Add a little water if needed to take it up to the MAX line.

6 Twist on the NUTRiBULLET blade and blend until smooth.

CHEF'S NOTE
Goji berries are high in antioxidants, vitamin C, iron & selenium.

HERB FRUIT BOOST

224 calories

Ingredients

- 75g/3oz pear
- 40g/1½oz avocado
- 150g/5oz cucumber
- 2 tsp lemon juice
- 1 tbsp coriander leaves
- 1 tbsp flat leaf parsley
- 1cm/½ inch fresh root ginger
- 120ml/ ½ cup coconut water
- Water

Method

1 Rinse the pear, cucumber, coriander and parsley. Core and roughly chop the pear. Chop the cucumber.

2 Add everything to the NUTRiBULLET tall cup. Make sure the ingredients do not go past the MAX line on your machine.

3 Add a little water if needed to take it up to the MAX line.

4 Twist on the NUTRiBULLET blade and blend until smooth.

CHEF'S NOTE
Coriander helps to build healthy skin and hair.

GRAPE & GREENS SMOOTHIE

240 calories

Ingredients

- 50g/2oz spinach
- 100g/3½oz pear
- 100g/3½oz seedless grapes
- 4 tbsp low fat Greek yoghurt

Method

1 Rinse the spinach, pear and grapes. Core the pear, but don't peel it.

2 Add everything to the NUTRiBULLET tall cup. Make sure the ingredients do not go past the MAX line on your machine.

3 Add a little water if needed to take it up to the MAX line.

4 Twist on the NUTRiBULLET blade and blend until smooth.

CHEF'S NOTE
Grapes have natural antioxidants called phytochemicals.

KIWI GREEN TEA SMOOTHIE

250 calories

Ingredients

ANTIOXIDANTS

- 250ml/1 cup green tea
- 150g/5oz kiwi
- 75g/3oz avocado
- 225g/8oz spinach
- A pinch of sea salt
- 1 tsp honey

Method

1 Make sure the green tea is no warmer than room temp.

2 Rinse the spinach well. Peel the kiwi. Peel and de-stone the avocado.

3 Add all the ingredients to the NUTRiBULLET tall cup. Make sure they don't go past the MAX line on your machine.

4 Twist on the NUTRiBULLET blade and blend until smooth.

CHEF'S NOTE
The many nutrients found in avocados are thought to help protect your body from heart disease, cancer and degenerative eye disease.

RASPBERRY & COCONUT OIL SMOOTHIE

291 calories

Ingredients

- 100g/3½oz raspberries
- 1 banana
- 225g/8oz spinach
- 1 tbsp coconut oil
- Water

Method

1 Wash the raspberries and the spinach well. Add them to the NUTRiBULLET tall cup.

2 Peel banana and add to the cup along with the coconut oil.

3 Fill to the MAX line with water.

4 Twist on the NUTRiBULLET blade and blend until smooth.

CHEF'S NOTE

Spinach is a superfood well known for its nutrients and health benefits to bones, eyes & digestion.

SPICY VEGETABLE SMOOTHIE

227 calories

Ingredients

GREEN GOODNESS

- 250ml/1 cup unsweetened almond milk
- 225g/8oz spinach
- 175g/6oz tomatoes
- Pinch sea salt
- Pinch cayenne pepper
- Water

Method

1 Rinse the spinach tomatoes and roughly chop.

2 Add the vegetables and almond milk to the NUTRiBULLET tall cup. Add the salt and Cayenne pepper. Make sure the ingredients do not go past the MAX line on your machine.

3 Add a little water if needed to take it up to the MAX line.

4 Twist on the NUTRiBULLET blade and blend until smooth.

CHEF'S NOTE

Nutribullet Tip....if you sometimes find your ingredients won't all fit in your cup under the max line. Try blending some together first to make room for the other ingredients.

KALE & DOUBLE SEED SMOOTHIE

298 calories

Ingredients

- 75g/3oz spinach
- 370ml/1½ cups almond milk
- 1 tbsp chia seeds
- 1 tbsp flax seeds
- Water

Method

1 Rinse the spinach and remove any thick stalks.

2 Add the spinach, almond milk & seeds to the NUTRiBULLET tall cup. Make sure the ingredients do not go past the MAX line on your machine.

3 Add a little water if needed to take it up to the MAX line.

4 Twist on the NUTRiBULLET blade and blend until smooth.

CHEF'S NOTE
This double blast of healthy seeds is packed with essential omega-3's.

HONEY ALMOND SMOOTHIE

262 calories

Ingredients

VITAMIN RICH

- 150g/5oz apple
- 150g/5oz orange
- 250ml/1 cup almond milk
- 1 tsp honey
- Water

Method

1 Rinse the ingredients well.

2 Peel and de-seed the orange.

3 Core the apple.

4 Add the fruit, honey & soya milk to the NUTRiBULLET tall cup. Make sure the ingredients do not go past the MAX line on your machine.

5 Add a little water if needed to take it up to the MAX line.

6 Twist on the NUTRiBULLET blade and blend until smooth.

CHEF'S NOTE
Almond milk works just as well for this fresh & bright smoothie.

AVOCADO & APPLE JUICE

295 calories

Ingredients

- 50g/2oz spinach
- 75g/3oz avocado
- 100g/3½oz apple
- 1 banana
- Water or ice

Method

1 Rinse the ingredients well.

2 Cut any thick stalks off the spinach

3 Peel & stone the avocado. Core the apple & peel the banana.

4 Add the vegetables & fruit to the NUTRiBULLET tall cup. Make sure the ingredients do not go past the MAX line on your machine.

5 Add water or ice, again being careful not to exceed the MAX line.

6 Twist on the NUTRiBULLET blade and blend until smooth.

CHEF'S NOTE

Avocado is a nutrient dense food that also adds luxurious smoothness to smoothies.

GREAT GREEN SMOOTHIE

205 calories

Ingredients

FIBRE SOURCE →

- 50g/2oz spinach
- 50g/2oz kale
- 125g/4oz asparagus
- 1 banana
- 1 tbsp chia seeds
- Water

Method

1 Rinse the ingredients well.

2 Cut any thick stalks off the kale and spinach

3 Peel the banana.

4 Add the vegetables, fruit & chia seeds to the NUTRiBULLET tall cup. Make sure the ingredients do not go past the MAX line on your machine.

5 Add water, again being careful not to exceed the MAX line.

6 Twist on the NUTRiBULLET blade and blend until smooth.

CHEF'S NOTE
Use only the sweet tips of the asparagus. Discard the thick woody ends.

ALMOND MILK & GINGER SMOOTHIE

245 calories

Ingredients

- 125g/4oz raspberries
- 250ml/1 cup unsweetened almond milk
- 50g/2oz pitted cherries
- 1½ tbsp honey
- 2 tsp fresh root ginger
- 2 tsp lemon juice
- Ice
- Water

Method

1 Wash the raspberries well and make sure all the cherries have been pitted.

2 Place all the ingredients in the NUTRiBULLET tall cup, finishing with ice.

3 Make sure the ingredients do not go past the MAX line on your machine.

4 Add a little water if needed to take it up to the MAX line.

5 Twist on the NUTRiBULLET blade and blend until smooth.

CHEF'S NOTE
Cherries contain natural aspirin that helps with inflammation issues.

SPIRULINA DETOX

295 calories

Ingredients

VITAMIN B +

- ½ small banana
- 50g/2oz blueberries
- 40g/1½oz avocado
- 120ml/ ½ cup unsweetened almond milk
- 1 tsp spirulina
- 1 tbsp almonds
- Water

Method

1 Rinse the berries. Peel the banana and the avocado. De-stone the avocado.

2 Add all the ingredients apart from water to the NUTRiBULLET tall cup. Make sure the ingredients do not go past the MAX line on your machine.

3 Add a little water if needed to take it up to the MAX line.

4 Twist on the NUTRiBULLET blade and blend until smooth.

CHEF'S NOTE
Spirulina is a form of blue-green algae with powerful healing and cleansing properties.

CRANBERRY & GREEN SMOOTHIE

292 calories

Ingredients

- 225g/8oz fresh kale
- 100g/3½oz fresh cranberries
- 140g/4½oz orange
- 1 banana
- 1 tbsp lime juice
- Water

Method

1 Rinse the kale and cranberries. Remove any thick stalks from the kale.

2 Peel and deseed the orange. Peel the banana and break into three.

3 Add all the ingredients to the NUTRiBULLET tall cup and top up with water to the MAX line on your machine.

4 Twist on the NUTRiBULLET blade and blend until smooth.

CHEF'S NOTE
Cranberries are high in fibre, vitamin C and manganese.

CREAMY BERRY & CHIA SMOOTHIE

297 calories

Ingredients

GOOD FATS ➤

- 75g/3oz avocado
- 50g/2oz fresh blueberries
- 1 tbsp chia seeds
- ¼ tsp cinnamon
- 2 tsp honey
- Water

Method

1 Rinse the blueberries well and place in the NUTRiBULLET tall cup.

2 Peel and de-stone the avocado.

3 Add the chia seeds, cinnamon and honey.

4 Add water to the MAX line on your machine.

5 Twist on the NUTRiBULLET blade and blend until smooth.

CHEF'S NOTE
Chia seeds are fabulously rich in omega 3, protein and antidioxidants.

COCONUT CREAM SMOOTHIE

255 calories

Ingredients

- 75g/3oz carrot
- 50g/2oz avocado
- 225g/8oz spinach

- 120ml/½ cup coconut water
- 1 tbsp coconut cream
- Ice cubes

Method

1 Rinse the spinach and carrot well.

2 Peel and stone the avocado.

3 Nip the ends of the carrots and place all the ingredients in the NUTRiBULLET tall cup, making sure they do not go past the MAX line on your machine.

4 Add the coconut water, cream and ice. Make sure the ingredients do not go past the MAX line on your machine.

5 Twist on the NUTRiBULLET blade and blend until smooth.

CHEF'S NOTE

Coconut water is a natural isotonic drink that provides many of the same benefits as formulated sports drinks, including calcium, magnesium, phosphorus, sodium and potassium.

BANANA & PINEAPPLE SMOOTHIE

288 calories

Ingredients

NATURALLY SWEET

- 400g/14oz fresh pineapple
- 1 small banana
- Ice cubes

Method

1 Peel the pineapple, cut it into chunks and drop into the NUTRiBULLET tall cup. Peel the banana, break it into three pieces and add.

2 Add ice to taste, but make sure the ingredients do not go past the MAX line on your machine.

3 Twist on the NUTRiBULLET blade and blend until smooth.

CHEF'S NOTE
Pineapple contains a wealth of nutrients including potassium, copper & manganese.

CITRUS SLUSHIE SMOOTHIE

253 calories

Ingredients

- 250g/9oz orange
- 125g/4oz raspberries
- 4 tbsp low fat natural Greek yoghurt
- Ice

Method

1 Rinse the raspberries well.

2 Peel & de-seed the orange.

3 Add everything to the NUTRiBULLET tall cup, making sure the ingredients do not go past the MAX line on your machine.

4 Twist on the NUTRiBULLET blade and blend until smooth.

CHEF'S NOTE
For extra sweetness add a teaspoon of agave nectar.

THE *Skinny*
NUTRiBULLET
LEAN BODY
ABS PLAN
NUTRIBLASTS UNDER 400 CALORIES

HONEY NUT SMOOTHIE

330 calories

Ingredients

SWEET & NUTTY

- 50g/2oz spinach
- 1 apple
- 1 banana
- 1 tbsp almonds
- 1 tbsp rolled oats
- 1 tbsp runny honey
- Water

Method

1 Rinse the ingredients well.

2 Core the apple, leaving the skin on. Peel the banana and break into three pieces.

3 Add the fruit, vegetables, oats & honey to the NUTRiBULLET tall cup. Make sure the ingredients do not go past the MAX line on your machine.

4 Add water, again being careful not to exceed the MAX line.

5 Twist on the NUTRiBULLET blade and blend until smooth.

CHEF'S NOTE
Use almond milk instead of water if you want a creamy finish.

SWEET PEPPER PICK UP JUICE

350 calories

Ingredients

- 50g/2oz spinach
- 1 yellow pepper
- 1 banana

- 200g/7oz fresh peeled pineapple
- Water

Method

1 Rinse the ingredients well.

2 Deseed the pepper, removing and discarding the stalk.

3 Peel the banana and break into three pieces.

4 Add all the fruit & vegetables to the NUTRiBULLET tall cup. Make sure the ingredients do not go past the MAX line on your machine.

5 Add water, again being careful not to exceed the MAX line.

6 Twist on the NUTRiBULLET blade and blend until smooth.

CHEF'S NOTE
Make sure you use a sweet ripe pepper for this juice.

ALMOND & ORANGE SMOOTHIE

350 calories

Ingredients

LIGHT & FRESH →

- 1 shredded romaine lettuce
- 2 oranges
- 125g/4oz carrot
- 1 tbsp chopped fresh mint
- 1 tbsp almonds
- 250ml/1 cup unsweetened almond milk
- Water

Method

1 Rinse the ingredients well.

2 Peel the oranges and separate into segments, don't worry about the pips.

3 Scrub the carrots, removing and discarding the tops before chopping.

4 Add all the fruit, vegetables, almonds & milk to the NUTRiBULLET tall cup. Make sure the ingredients do not go past the MAX line on your machine.

5 Add water, again being careful not to exceed the MAX line.

6 Twist on the NUTRiBULLET blade and blend until smooth.

CHEF'S NOTE
Optional Nutriboost: Add 1 tablespoon of protein powder.

SWEET COCONUT JUICE

393 calories

Ingredients

- 50g/2oz spinach
- 1 banana
- 200g/7oz fresh peeled pineapple
- 250ml/1 cup coconut water

Method

1 Rinse the ingredients well.

2 Peel the banana and break into three pieces.

3 Add the fruit, vegetables & coconut water to the NUTRiBULLET tall cup. Make sure the ingredients do not go past the MAX line on your machine.

4 Twist on the NUTRiBULLET blade and blend until smooth.

CHEF'S NOTE
Use as much coconut water as you need to reach the max line.

CASHEW CLEANSE

393 calories

Ingredients

GOOD FATS →

- 50g/2oz spinach
- 1 banana
- 75g/3oz fresh peeled pineapple
- 250ml/1 cup unsweetened almond milk
- 10 fresh cashew nuts
- Water

Method

1 Rinse the ingredients well.

2 Peel the banana and break each into three pieces.

3 Add all the fruit, vegetables, nuts & milk to the NUTRiBULLET tall cup. Make sure the ingredients do not go past the MAX line on your machine.

4 Add water, again being careful not to exceed the MAX line.

5 Twist on the NUTRiBULLET blade and blend until smooth.

CHEF'S NOTE
Optional Nutriboost: Add 1 teaspoon of flax or chia seeds.

LIME & CRANBERRY SMOOTHIE

301 calories

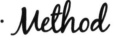

Ingredients

- 1 shredded romaine lettuce
- 1 apple
- ½ lime
- 1 banana
- 200g/7oz fresh cranberries
- Water

Method

1 Rinse the ingredients well.

2 Core the apple, leaving the skin on. Peel the lime, don't worry about the pips.

3 Add all the fruit & vegetables to the NUTRiBULLET tall cup. Make sure the ingredients do not go past the MAX line on your machine.

4 Add water, again being careful not to exceed the MAX line.

5 Twist on the NUTRiBULLET blade and blend until smooth.

CHEF'S NOTE
Optional Nutriboost: Add 1 tablespoon of acai berries.

SUPER GREEN MILK SMOOTHIE

305 calories

Ingredients

GOOD & GREEN

- 50g/2oz kale
- 1 courgette
- ½ cucumber
- 1 apple
- 1 pear
- 250ml/1 cup semi skimmed milk
- Water

Method

1 Rinse the ingredients well.

2 Remove any thick stalks from the kale.

3 Top and tail the courgette & cucumber, leaving the skin on.

4 Core the apple, leaving the skin on.

5 Add all the fruit, vegetables & milk to the NUTRiBULLET tall cup. Make sure the ingredients do not go past the MAX line on your machine.

6 Add water, again being careful not to exceed the MAX line.

7 Twist on the NUTRiBULLET blade and blend until smooth.

CHEF'S NOTE
Try adding some lemon too.

TURMERIC CLEANSER

305 calories

Ingredients

- 50g/2oz spinach
- 150g/5oz carrots
- 1 banana

- ½ tsp turmeric
- 250ml/1 cup soya milk
- Water

Method

1 Rinse the ingredients well.

2 Scrub the carrots, discarding the tops before chopping.

3 Peel the banana and break into three pieces.

4 Add the fruit, vegetables, turmeric & milk to the NUTRiBULLET tall cup. Make sure the ingredients do not go past the MAX line on your machine.

5 Add water, again being careful not to exceed the MAX line.

6 Twist on the NUTRiBULLET blade and blend until smooth.

CHEF'S NOTE

Turmeric is often used in traditional medicines however it can stain cooking equipment, so make sure you wash everything straight away.

SWEET POTATO SOYA SMOOTHIE

305 calories

Ingredients

ROOT GOODNESS

- 50g/2oz spinach
- 150g/5oz sweet potatoes
- Pinch of ground nutmeg
- 250ml/1 cup soya milk
- 1 tsp runny honey
- Water

Method

1 Rinse the ingredients well.

2 Cube the sweet potatoes, leaving the skin on.

3 Add the vegetables, nutmeg, milk & honey to the NUTRiBULLET tall cup. Make sure the ingredients do not go past the MAX line on your machine.

4 Add water (if there's space), again being careful not to exceed the MAX line.

5 Twist on the NUTRiBULLET blade and blend until smooth.

CHEF'S NOTE
Optional Nutriboost: Add 1 tablespoon of shelled fresh walnuts.

FLAX SEED & BERRY BLAST

310 calories

Ingredients

- 50g/2oz spinach
- 1 banana
- 250g/9oz strawberries
- 1 tbsp flax seeds
- 250ml/1 cup unsweetened almond milk
- Water

Method

1 Rinse the ingredients well.

2 Peel the banana and break into three pieces.

3 Cut the green tops of the strawberries.

4 Add all the fruit & vegetables to the NUTRiBULLET tall cup. Make sure the ingredients do not go past the MAX line on your machine.

5 Add water, again being careful not to exceed the MAX line.

6 Twist on the NUTRiBULLET blade and blend until smooth.

CHEF'S NOTE
Any berries work well in this power packed smoothie.

SALAD & BANANA BLASTER

320 calories

Ingredients

TRY ALMOND MILK →

- 1 shredded romaine lettuce
- 1 pear
- 1 banana
- 250ml/1 cup semi skimmed milk
- Water

Method

1 Rinse the ingredients well.

2 Core the pear, leaving the skin on. Peel the banana and break into three pieces.

3 Add all the fruit, lettuce and milk to the NUTRiBULLET tall cup. Make sure the ingredients do not go past the MAX line on your machine.

4 Add water, again being careful not to exceed the MAX line.

5 Twist on the NUTRiBULLET blade and blend until smooth.

CHEF'S NOTE
Optional Nutriboost: Add 1 tablespoon of acai berries.

LEMON & GINGER SOYA SMOOTHIE

380 calories

Ingredients

- 50g/2oz spinach
- ½ lemon
- 1 banana
- 150g/5oz fresh peeled pineapple
- 2cm/1 inch fresh ginger root
- 250ml/1 cup soya milk
- Water

Method

1 Rinse the ingredients well.

2 Peel the lemon, don't worry about the pips. Peel the banana and break into three pieces.

3 Add all the fruit, vegetables and milk to the NUTRiBULLET tall cup. Make sure the ingredients do not go past the MAX line on your machine.

4 Add water, again being careful not to exceed the MAX line.

5 Twist on the NUTRiBULLET blade and blend until smooth.

CHEF'S NOTE
Optional Nutriboost: Add 1 teaspoon of hemp seeds.

PUMPKIN CARROT PROTEIN SHAKE

370 calories

Ingredients

MUSCLE BUILDER

- 50g/2oz spinach
- 150g/5oz carrots
- 200g/7oz mixed berries
- 120ml/½ cup almond milk
- 1 tbsp pumpkin seeds
- 1 scoop protein powder
- Water

Method

1 Rinse the ingredients well.

2 Scrub and slice the carrots, discarding the tops.

3 Add the fruit, vegetables, pumpkin seeds, protein powder & almond milk to the NUTRiBULLET tall cup. Make sure the ingredients do not go past the MAX line on your machine.

4 Add water, (if there is space) again being careful not to exceed the MAX line.

5 Twist on the NUTRiBULLET blade and blend until smooth.

CHEF'S NOTE
Optional Nutriboost: Add 1 tablespoon of goji berries seeds.

KALE & FRUIT COCONUT WATER

302 calories

Ingredients

- 50g/2oz kale
- 1 celery stalk
- 125g/4oz apple

- 1 banana
- 200g/7oz fresh pineapple
- 250ml/1 cup coconut water

Method

1 Rinse the ingredients well.

2 Remove any thick stalks from the kale.

3 Chop the celery stalk. Peel the banana and break into three pieces.

4 Core the apple, leaving the skin on.

5 Add all the ingredients to the NUTRiBULLET tall cup. Making sure they do not go past the MAX line on your machine.

6 Twist on the NUTRiBULLET blade and blend until smooth.

CHEF'S NOTE
A spoonful of coconut cream makes a good addition.

FRUITY FLAX SEED SMOOTHIE

360 calories

Ingredients

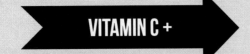

VITAMIN C +

- 50g/2oz spinach
- 75g/3oz kiwi fruit
- 175g/6oz fresh mango
- 1 banana
- 100g/3½oz carrots
- 2 tsp of flax seeds
- Water

Method

1 Rinse the ingredients well.

2 Peel & dice the kiwi. De-stone and peel the mango. Peel the banana and break into three pieces.

3 Scrub the carrot. Remove the top and slice.

4 Add the fruit, vegetables & flax seeds to the NUTRiBULLET tall cup. Make sure the ingredients do not go past the MAX line on your machine.

5 Add water, again being careful not to exceed the MAX line.

6 Twist on the NUTRiBULLET blade and blend until smooth.

CHEF'S NOTE
Try with coconut water too.

PEAR & ALMOND YOGURT SMOOTHIE

335 calories

Ingredients

- 1 tbsp almonds
- 100g/3½oz apple
- 1 banana
- 2 tbsp low fat Greek yoghurt
- 250ml/1 cup unsweetened almond milk
- ½ tsp ground cinnamon
- Water

Method

1 Rinse and core the apple.

2 Peel the banana and break into three pieces.

3 Add all the ingredients to the NUTRiBULLET tall cup. Make sure they do not go past the MAX line on your machine.

4 Add a little water if needed to take it up to the MAX line.

5 Twist on the NUTRiBULLET blade and blend until smooth.

CHEF'S NOTE
Almonds contain useful antioxidants which cleanse toxins.

BLUEBERRY COCONUT MILK

310 calories

Ingredients

FRUITY

- 100g/3½oz blueberries
- 180ml/¾ cup light coconut milk
- A pinch of ground cinnamon
- 1 tsp honey
- 1 tbsp chia seeds
- Water

Method

1 Rinse the blueberries. Add them to the NUTRiBULLET tall cup, along with the other ingredients, making sure not go past the MAX line on your machine.

2 Add a little water if needed to take it up to the MAX line.

3 Twist on the NUTRiBULLET blade and blend until smooth.

CHEF'S NOTE
Chia seeds contain high amounts of both soluble and insoluble fibre, and help to clean out the digestive tract.

AVOCADO CACAO SMOOTHIE

305 calories

Ingredients

- 250ml/1 cup coconut water
- 100g/3 ½oz avocado
- 75g/3oz raspberries
- 1 tbsp cacao powder
- 75g/3oz spinach

Method

1 Rinse the raspberries and spinach well.

2 Peel and de-stone the avocado.

3 Add all the ingredients to the NUTRiBULLET tall cup. Make sure they don't go past the MAX line on your machine.

4 Twist on the NUTRiBULLET blade and blend until smooth.

CHEF'S NOTE
Raw cacao contains nearly four times the antioxidant content of processed dark chocolate.

CARROT & RAISIN NUT SMOOTHIE

399 calories

Ingredients

HIGH ENERGY ➤

- 75g/3oz avocado
- 50g/2oz carrot
- 3 tbsp raisins
- 125g/4oz spinach
- 250ml/1 cup unsweetened almond milk
- ½ tsp cinnamon
- Water

Method

1 Wash the carrot and spinach. Nip the ends off the carrot.

2 Peel and de-stone the avocado.

3 Add everything to the NUTRiBULLET tall cup. Make sure the ingredients do not go past the MAX line on your machine.

4 Top up with water if needed to take it up to the MAX line.

5 Twist on the NUTRiBULLET blade and blend until smooth.

CHEF'S NOTE

Almond milk is low in fat and high in energy, proteins, lipids and fibre.

BANANA SOYA MILK

340 calories

Ingredients

- 2 bananas
- 3 tbsp low-fat vanilla yogurt
- 120ml/½ cup soya milk

- 1 tsp honey
- Pinch of ground cinnamon
- Ice

Method

1 Peel the bananas and break each into three pieces.

2 Add everything to the NUTRiBULLET tall cup, finishing with ice. Make sure you don't go past the MAX line on your machine.

3 Twist on the NUTRiBULLET blade and blend until smooth.

CHEF'S NOTE
Experiment with more cinnamon for a warmer, spicier taste.

Abs Plan WORKOUTS

Toning and building muscle in your core takes work and yes it can be tough. For the first few day you will likely suffer from tight and tender muscles in your abdominals but as you regularly exercise, this will ease and you will be able to focus on getting the best from your workouts.

We have compiled **4** core workouts to perform throughout each week. Choose one workout to perform per day and use the remaining 3 days to rest. Try to alternate between training and rest days. Each workout lasts for approximately 15 mins and a simple explanation of how to correctly perform each exercise in the set is explained in the following pages.

It is very important to warm up your muscles and joints before beginning any exercise to prevent injury and to make sure you perform each repetition to the best of your ability. Warm up by jogging on the spot for two minutes. Stand upright, with your feet shoulder-width apart. Contract and release your abdominal muscles for 15 to 20 repetitions to warm up your abs.

Always cool down and stretch at the end of your workout. Gently jog for 2 minutes then stretch out your core by performing the cobra and cat & cow stretches. (see page 94).

Tips

· Warm up and cool down before and after each workout

· Have a bottle of water to drink from between sets

· Remember to breathe through each exercise

· Keep your core tight

Core WORKOUT ONE

- Exercise 1: **BICYCLE CRUNCH** 30 secs | 10 secs rest
- Exercise 2: **LEG RAISE** 30 secs | 10 secs rest
- Exercise 3: **STANDING SIDE CRUNCH** 30 secs | 10 secs rest
- Exercise 4: **T STABILASTION** 30 secs | 10 secs rest
- Exercise 5: **JUMPING JACK** Hold position for 15 secs then reverse position for a further 15 secs | 10 secs rest
- Exercise 6: **V – UP** 30 secs | 2 minute rest

Repeat for 2 more sets

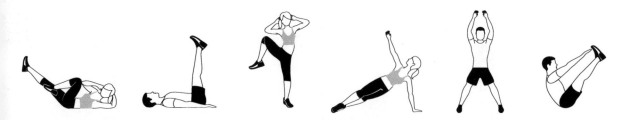

Perform each exercise as many times as possible within 30 seconds or hold for the desired length of time depending on the drill. Rest for 10 seconds then perform the next exercise again for 30 secs with a 10 sec rest in between exercises. Repeat until all 6 exercises have been completed.

Rest for 2 minutes then repeat the whole set two more times with a 2 minute rest in between.

Bicycle CRUNCH

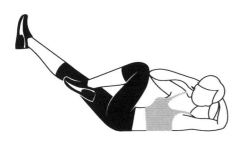 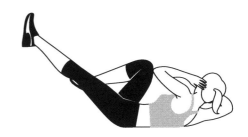

Lie face up and place your hands behind your head, supporting your neck with your fingers. Make sure your core is tight and the small of your back is pushed hard against the floor. Lift your knees in toward your chest while lifting your shoulder blades off the floor. Rotate to the right, bringing the left elbow towards the right knee as you extend the other leg into the air. Switch sides, bringing the right elbow towards the left knee. Alternate each side in a pedalling motion.

Leg RAISE

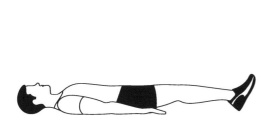 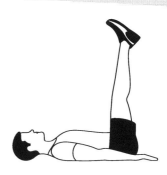

Lie on your back. Place your hands, palms down, on the floor beside you. Raise your legs off the ground (exhale as you go) until your toes are pointing to the ceiling and your legs are straight. Keep your knees locked throughout the exercise. Hold for 2 secs then lower your legs to approximately 6 inches from the floor before raising then again.

Standing SIDE CRUNCH

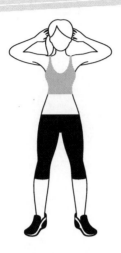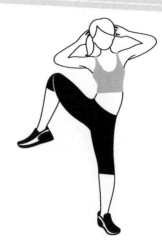

Stand with feet shoulder-width apart, core engaged and knees slightly bent. Lift your right leg, bending the knee 90 degrees and turning thigh out to side. Place both hands behind your head and crunch your right elbow to your right knee. Alternate between legs.

T-STABILISATION

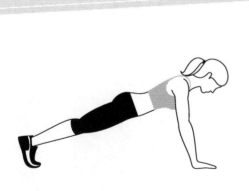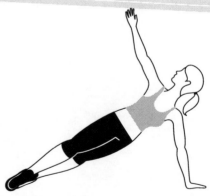

Assume a standard push-up position. Lift your right arm up as you rotate your body to the right using your right leg to cross your left for balance. Rotate all the way over until your arm is straight up and your left side is facing the ground. Your body will now look like a "T" on its side. Hold this position for 5 secs. Reverse movements back to starting position. Repeat on opposite side.

Jumping JACKS

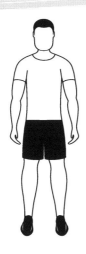 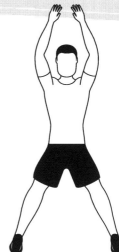

Stand with your feet together and your hands down by your side. In one motion jump your feet out to the side and raise your arms above your head. Immediately reverse by jumping back to the starting position.

V-UP

 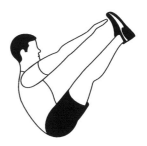

Lay flat on the floor with your legs straight and your arms extended over your head. Lift your chest and legs up off the ground in unison. Your chest should be led by your arms. You should aim to touch your toes at the top of each repetition. As you touch your toes, the top of your tail bone should be the only thing in contact with the ground.

Core WORKOUT TWO

- Exercise 1: **SIT UP** 30 secs | 10 secs rest
- Exercise 2: **FLUTTER KICK** 30 secs | 10 secs rest
- Exercise 3: **WINDSHIELD WIPERS** 30 secs | 10 secs rest
- Exercise 4: **MOUNTAIN CLIMBER** 30 secs | 10 secs rest
- Exercise 5: **SUPERMAN** 30 secs | 10 secs rest
- Exercise 6: **PLANK JACK** 30 secs | 2 minute rest

Repeat for 2 more sets

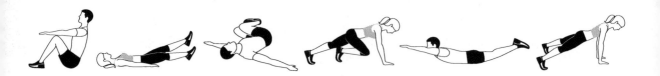

Perform each exercise as many times as possible within 30 seconds or hold for the desired length of time depending on the drill. Rest for 10 seconds then perform the next exercise again for 30 secs with a 10 sec rest in between exercises. Repeat until all 6 exercises have been completed.

Rest for 2 minutes then repeat the whole set two more times with a 2 minute rest in between.

Sit UP

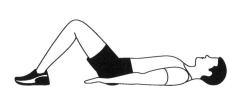 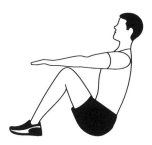

Lie on your back with your knees bent and your arms extended at your sides. and your feet flat on the floor. Engage your core and slowly curl your upper back off the floor towards your knees with your arms extended out. Roll back down to the starting position.

Flutter KICK

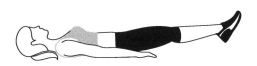 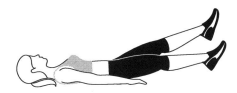

Lie on your back with legs straight and extend your arms by your sides. Lift your heels about 6 inches and quickly kick your feet up and down in a scissor-like motion.

Windshield WIPERS

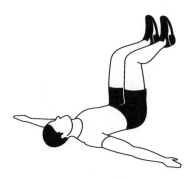 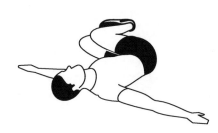

Lie on your back with your arms straight out to the sides. Lift your legs and bend the knees at a 90-degree angle. Rotate the hips to one side without letting the legs touch the floor. Lift your legs and return to the starting position. Rotate the hips to the opposite side and repeat.

Mountain CLIMBER

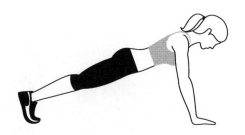 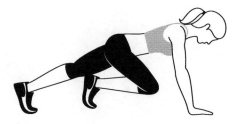

Begin in a pushup position, with your weight supported by your hands and toes. Flexing the knee and hip, bring one leg towards the corresponding arm. Explosively reverse the positions of your legs, extending the bent leg until the leg is straight and supported by the toe, and bringing the other foot up with the hip and knee flexed. Repeat in an alternating fashion.

Superman

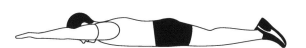 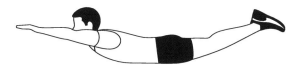

Lie straight and face down on the floor. Simultaneously raise your arms, legs, and chest off of the floor and hold this position for 2 seconds. Slowly begin to lower your arms, legs and chest back down to the starting position while inhaling.

Plank JACK

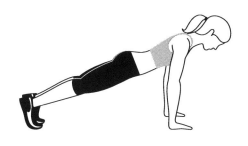 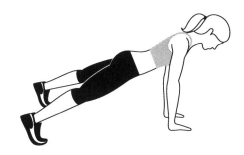

Start in the plank position with more weight resting on your forearms. The body should form a straight line from the shoulders to the ankles. Engage your core then jump the feet out to the sides as if you were performing a jumping jack but keep the upper body still. Return to the starting position and repeat.

Core WORKOUT THREE

- Exercise 1: **PULSE UPS** 30 secs | 10 secs rest
- Exercise 2: **REVERSE PLANK** 30 secs | 10 secs rest
- Exercise 3: **HIGH KNEES** 30 secs | 10 secs rest
- Exercise 4: **RUSSIAN TWIST** 30 secs | 10 secs rest
- Exercise 5: **L SIT** Hold position for as long as possible | start with 2 sec holds | 10 secs rest
- Exercise 6: **SIDE PLANK LEG LIFT** 15 secs on each side | 2 minute rest

- **Repeat for 2 more sets**

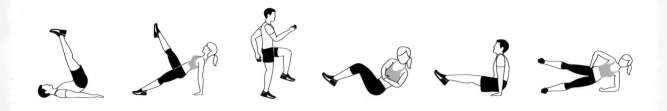

Perform each exercise as many times as possible within 30 seconds or hold for the desired length of time depending on the drill. Rest for 10 seconds then perform the next exercise again for 30 secs with a 10 sec rest in between exercises. Repeat until all 6 exercises have been completed.

Rest for 2 minutes then repeat the whole set two more times with a 2 minute rest in between.

Pulse **UPS**

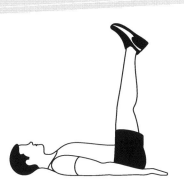 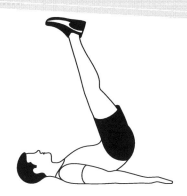

Lie flat on the ground and place your hands at your sides. Raise your legs vertically upwards so that that they are perpendicular to the floor. Start raising your upper body by contracting your core and reaching out for the legs. Feel a squeeze in your abdominal muscles and glutes. Return to the starting position.

Reverse **PLANK**

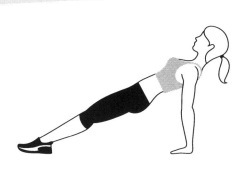 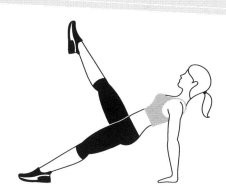

Sit tall with both your legs extended. Place your hands flat to the floor behind you, fingers facing in. Press into your hands and feet to raise your torso, forming a straight line from your head lo your loes. Lift your right leg to the ceiling and hold for 3 secs. Return your right leg to the floor then lift the leg leg again holding for 3 secs in raised position.

High KNEES

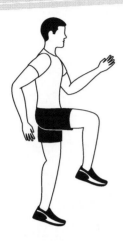 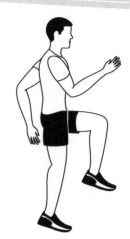

Stand straight with the feet hip width apart, looking straight ahead and arms hanging down by your side. Jump from one foot to the other at the same time lifting your knees as high as possible, hip height is advisable. The arms should be following the motion. Try holding your hands just above the hips so that your knees touch the palms of your hands as you lift your knees.

Russian TWIST

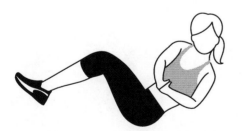 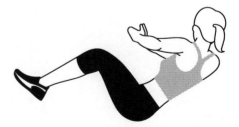

Sit on the floor with your hips and knees bent 90 degrees with arms extended and hands clasped and your back straight (your torso should be at about 45 degrees to the floor). Explosively twist your torso as far as you can to the left and then reverse the motion, twisting as far as you can to the right.

ℒ-SIT

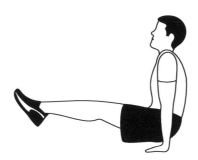

Sit on the floor with your hands directly under your shoulders, fingers facing forward. From this position, push into the floor with your hands, straighten your arms, and bring your shoulders down in order to lift your tail bone off the floor. Hold this position. Begin by holding for just a few seconds then as you grow stronger, progress to longer periods aiming for 15-30 second holds.

Side Plank LEG LIFT

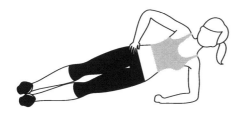 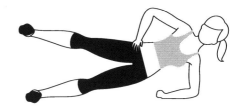

Place your left elbow on the ground. Keeping your spine lengthened and your abs engaged, lift your right leg up just higher than your top hip. Keep your waist up and lifted, and don't let your upper body drop in to your bottom shoulder. Return your leg to the starting position. Repeat for 15 seconds then change position so your right elbow is on the ground lifting your left leg.

Core WORKOUT FOUR

- Exercise 1: **BIRD DOG** 30 secs | 10 secs rest
- Exercise 2: **SPIDERMAN PLANK** 30 secs | 10 secs rest
- Exercise 3: **WALL SIT** Hold for up to 30 secs | 10 secs rest
- Exercise 4: **SIDE PLANK CRUNCH** 15 secs on each side | 10 secs rest
- Exercise 5: **SIDE SKATER** 30 secs | 10 secs rest
- Exercise 6: **REVERSE CRUNCH** 30 secs | 2 minute rest

Repeat for 2 more sets

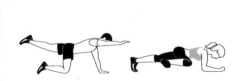 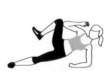

Perform each exercise as many times as possible within 30 seconds or hold for the desired length of time depending on the drill. Rest for 10 seconds then perform the next exercise again for 30 secs with a 10 sec rest in between exercises. Repeat until all 6 exercises have been completed.

Rest for 2 minutes then repeat the whole set two more times with a 2 minute rest in between.

Bird DOG

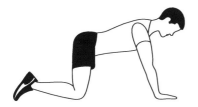 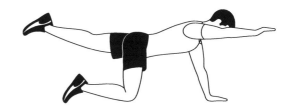

Begin on all fours, knees hip-width apart and under the hips, hands flat and shoulder-width apart. Squeeze your abs by pulling belly toward spine. Keep the spine in a neutral position and extend your left leg back and your right arm straight ahead. Hold for two to three seconds then reverse position to extend your right leg and left arm.

Spiderman PLANK

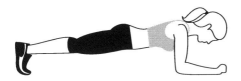 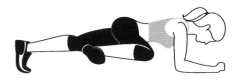

Start in a traditional plank position with your forearms on the ground and your body straight. Bring your right knee forward towards your right elbow, then return to the extended plank position. Repeat by bringing your left knee toward your left elbow.

Wall SIT

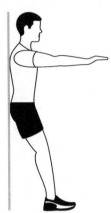 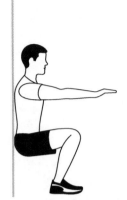

Lean against the wall with your feet planted firmly on the ground, shoulder width apart and approximately two feet away from the wall. Slowly slide down the wall with your back pressed against it until your legs are bent at a 90 degree angle. Your knees should also be directly above your ankles and your back should be touching the wall at all times. Hold the position for as long as possible up to 30 secs.

Side Plank CRUNCH

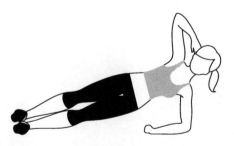 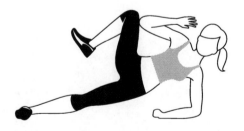

Begin in a side elbow plank position with your left elbow on the ground and your right hand behind your head. Keeping your spine lengthened and with your core engaged, bring your right leg up toward your shoulder to lightly tap your right elbow. Straighten your right leg back to the starting position. Repeat for 10 seconds then change position so your right elbow is on the ground lifting your left leg to the left elbow. Repeat for another 10 seconds.

Side SKATER

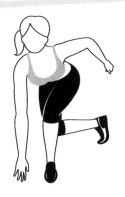 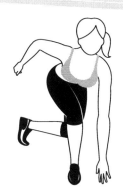

Start in a squat position with your left leg bent at the knee and your right arm parallel for balance. Your right leg is extended but still bent at the knee behind you. Jump sideways to the right, landing on your right leg. Bring your left leg behind you with your left arm extended and fingers touching the floor. Keep your back straight and your core engaged. Reverse direction by jumping to the left.

Reverse CRUNCH

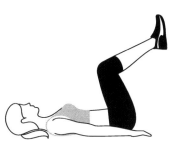 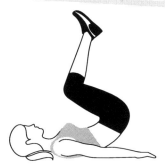

Lie on your back and extend your arms out to the side. Raise your knees and feet so they create a 90-degree angle. Contract your abdominals and exhale as you lift your hips off the floor. Your knees will move toward your head. Try to keep your knees at a right angle. Inhale and slowly lower.

Cobra STRETCH

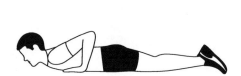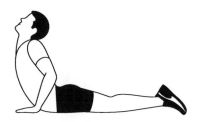

Lay on your stomach with your palms facing down and positioned right underneath your shoulders. Keep your legs shoulder-width apart. Pushing down with your hands, lift your chest as you exhale. Be sure to keep your hips and the tops of your feet firmly planted on the floor. You should feel a rewarding stretch in your core. Slowly lower your chest back to floor. Repeat 5 times.

Cat Cow STRETCH

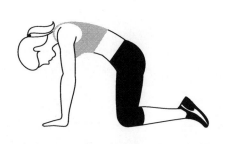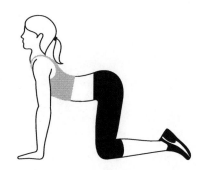

Begin with your hands and knees on the floor. Exhale while rounding your spine up towards the ceiling, pulling your belly button up towards your spine, and engaging your core. Inhale while arching your back and letting your tummy relax. Repeat 5 times.

Printed in Great Britain
by Amazon